Science of Sleep

Decoding Dreamland

John Ray

TScience of Sleep: Decoding Dreamland

John Ray

Table of Content

Introduction

What is Sleep

Sleep is a state of recurring behavioral rest, characterized by several characteristics, such as reduced awareness of and response to stimuli, decreased consciousness, and a rhythmic manifestation of physiologic states (stages). It tends to occur at particular parts of the 24-hour day–night cycle, and at customary locations, both depending on the particular species and environment. It is reversible, distinguishing it from coma or ongoing anesthesia. It is also self-regulating: if one is deprived of sleep, there will be a drive to have increased "recovery sleep" to make up for the loss.

THE BENEFITS OF SLEEP

Sleep is beneficial for mind, body, and spirit. Getting the right amount of good-quality sleep is one of the most effective self-help measures you can take to maintain or regain your health and boost your sense of well-being. Here are just a few of the advantages that sleeping well can bring you:

- Physical Restoration and Healing: Sleep serves as a vital time for the body to repair and regenerate. Deep sleep stages result in tissue and muscle regeneration, as well as a strengthening of the immune system. This restoration process is essential for overall physical health and longevity.

- Cognitive Function and Memory Consolidation: Adequate sleep is integral to cognitive functions such as memory consolidation, learning, and problem-solving. It enhances the brain's ability to organize and store information, facilitating improved concentration and mental clarity.

- Emotional Well-being: Sleep has a profound impact on emotional regulation and stability.

Insufficient sleep can contribute to irritability, mood swings, and an increased susceptibility to stress. On the other hand, quality sleep supports emotional resilience and helps maintain a positive outlook.

- Metabolic Balance and Weight Regulation: Sleep plays a crucial role in regulating hormones that control appetite and metabolism. Lack of sleep disrupts this balance, leading to increased hunger and a higher likelihood of weight gain. Adequate sleep is, therefore, a key component of maintaining a healthy weight.

- Cardiovascular Health: Chronic sleep deprivation has been linked to an increased risk of cardiovascular diseases, including hypertension and heart attacks. Quality sleep contributes to the maintenance of a healthy cardiovascular system by allowing the heart and blood vessels to rest and recuperate.

- Hormonal Regulation: Sleep is intricately connected to the regulation of various hormones, including those that influence growth, stress response, and reproductive functions. Consistent and restful sleep supports the proper functioning of these hormonal systems.

- Enhanced Creativity and Problem-Solving: Adequate sleep has been shown to enhance creativity and improve problem-solving skills. It allows the brain to make connections between seemingly unrelated information, fostering innovation and ingenuity.

- Improved Mood and Stress Management: Sleep has a direct impact on mood regulation, and a lack of it can contribute to increased stress levels. Conversely, a well-rested mind is better equipped to handle stress and maintain emotional balance.

- Enhanced Physical Performance: Athletes recognize the importance of sleep in optimizing physical performance. Restorative sleep contributes to improved muscle recovery, coordination, and overall athletic prowess.

- Long-term Cognitive Health: Adequate and quality sleep has been associated with a lower risk of cognitive decline and neurodegenerative conditions in later life. It is considered a protective factor for long-term brain health.

EFFECT OF INSUFFICIENT SLEEP

Insufficient sleep can have a multitude of detrimental effects on both physical and mental well-being. The negative impact of not getting enough sleep extends beyond mere tiredness and can manifest in various aspects of daily life.

- Cognitive Functioning: One of the most apparent consequences of inadequate sleep is impaired cognitive function. Memory consolidation, problem-solving abilities, and overall cognitive performance suffer when the brain is deprived of the rest it needs. This can result in difficulty concentrating, decreased alertness, and slower reaction times.

- Mood Disturbances: Sleep plays a crucial role in regulating mood. Insufficient sleep is linked to increased irritability, mood swings, and heightened stress levels. Prolonged lack of adequate sleep has been linked to an increased likelihood of developing depressive and anxiety-related mood disorders.

- Physical Health: The body undergoes essential repair and maintenance processes during sleep. Not getting enough rest compromises the immune system, making individuals more susceptible to illnesses. Moreover, chronic sleep deprivation is linked to an increased risk of conditions like obesity, diabetes, and cardiovascular diseases.

- Impaired Motor Skills: Sleep deprivation can have a profound impact on motor skills and coordination. This poses serious risks, especially for those who need to operate machinery or drive vehicles. The likelihood of accidents and errors significantly increases when individuals are sleep-deprived.

- Decreased Productivity: The ability to perform tasks efficiently and effectively is compromised when sleep is insufficient. This can lead to decreased productivity at work or in academic settings. It hampers creativity, problem-solving skills, and the capacity to make sound decisions.

- Weight Gain and Metabolic Disruptions: Lack of sleep disrupts the balance of hormones that regulate appetite. This disruption can lead to increased cravings for high-calorie foods, contributing to weight gain. Additionally, insufficient sleep affects insulin sensitivity, potentially increasing the risk of developing metabolic disorders.

- Impact on Relationships: Sleep deprivation can strain relationships. Irritability and mood swings resulting from lack of sleep can lead to conflicts with friends, family, and colleagues. Furthermore, the overall stress caused by sleep deprivation can affect communication and emotional well-being.

- Compromised Safety: Fatigue due to lack of sleep poses a significant risk to safety. In professions that require high levels of alertness, such as healthcare, transportation, or emergency services, the consequences of impaired attention and reaction times can be severe.

STAGES OF SLEEP

When a person is asleep, their brain goes through four different sleep stages. The first three stages are called NREM sleep, which is a gradually deeper sleep. The last stage is called rapid eye movement sleep, which is more of a dream-like state. The body goes through each stage about 4 to 6 times during a night.

Stage 1 NREM (Light sleep)

Stage 1 of Non-Rapid Eye Movement (NREM) sleep, often referred to as Light Sleep, marks the initial phase of the sleep cycle. This stage serves as a transitional period as an individual moves from the wakeful state to a deeper sleep. During Stage 1, various physiological changes take place, contributing to the overall relaxation and preparation for more profound sleep stages.

One significant characteristic of Stage 1 NREM sleep is the attenuation of brain activity. The brain waves gradually shift from the faster patterns of wakefulness to slower, more synchronized waves. This alteration in brain wave activity is accompanied by a reduction in heart rate, a slowing of the respiratory rate, and a decrease in eye movements. These collective changes signify the body's descent into a state of rest.

Muscle relaxation is another notable feature of Stage 1. As the body eases into the initial throes of sleep, muscles start to loosen and unwind. Although not completely devoid of muscle activity, there may be occasional twitches or jerks during this stage. These sporadic movements are normal and are often referred to as hypnic jerks.

It's important to note that Stage 1 NREM sleep is relatively brief. Individuals typically spend only a small percentage of their total sleep time in this initial stage, approximately around 5%. The brevity of Stage 1 makes it a transient phase, paving the way for the subsequent stages of NREM sleep and eventually leading into the more restorative Rapid Eye Movement (REM) sleep.

Stage 1 NREM sleep is a crucial gateway between wakefulness and deeper sleep. It orchestrates a symphony of physiological changes, from the slowing of brain waves and vital signs to the relaxation of muscles, setting the stage for the more profound and rejuvenating sleep to come.

Stage 2 NREM (Deeper sleep)

During Stage 2 of NREM (Non-Rapid Eye Movement) sleep, the transition into deeper slumber takes a more pronounced hold on the individual. As the body succumbs to the embrace of rest, there is a discernible decline in physiological activity. The heart rate continues its descent, easing into a slower, more rhythmic pace. Muscles, too, relinquish their tension, allowing a profound state of relaxation to permeate the entire body.

One prominent feature of Stage 2 NREM sleep is the further descent of body temperature. This cooling effect contributes to the overall physiological changes, facilitating a conducive environment for the body to regenerate and rejuvenate during the restorative sleep process. Intriguingly, during this stage, a remarkable phenomenon occurs—eye movements come to a temporary standstill. This cessation of ocular activity is in stark contrast to the rapid eye movements observed during REM sleep phases.

As the body surrenders to deeper slumber, the brain-wave activity undergoes a noteworthy transformation. While it slows down overall, there are intermittent bursts of electrical activity termed "sleep spindles." These fleeting surges of neural energy, characterized by their distinctive spindle-shaped waveform, play a crucial role in the consolidation of memories. Studies suggest that these sleep spindles contribute significantly to the encoding and retention of information, assisting in the optimization of memory functions.

Interestingly, individuals spend a substantial portion of their total sleep time in Stage 2 NREM, accounting for approximately 45% of the sleep cycle. This prolonged duration underscores the importance of this stage in the overall sleep architecture. During the initial cycle, Stage 2 typically spans around 25 minutes, with the duration gradually extending in subsequent cycles.

In essence, Stage 2 NREM sleep signifies a pivotal juncture in the intricate tapestry of the sleep cycle. As the body and mind undergo a series of orchestrated changes, from the slackening of muscles to the dance of sleep spindles in the neural landscape, this stage sets the foundation for the deeper phases of restorative sleep that follow.

Stage 3 NREM (Deepest sleep)

Stage 3 NREM, often referred to as the Deepest Sleep or Slow-Wave Sleep (SWS), is a critical phase in the sleep cycle, constituting approximately 25% of the entire sleep duration. During this stage, various physiological processes undergo profound changes, contributing to the rejuvenation and maintenance of overall health.

In Stage 3 NREM, a person experiences a significant decrease in heart rate, breathing rate, and brain wave activity. These vital signs reach their lowest levels, signifying a state of deep and restorative sleep. Simultaneously, the muscles in the body reach a state of complete relaxation. This deep relaxation makes this stage particularly challenging to awaken from, and it is during this phase that certain sleep-related phenomena, such as sleepwalking, bedwetting, and night terrors, may manifest.

One of the primary functions of Stage 3 NREM is the promotion of physical restoration and repair. During this stage, the body engages in essential processes such as the repair of tissues, the strengthening of the immune system, and the regeneration of bone and muscle. These reparative activities are crucial for overall well-being and contribute to the maintenance of optimal health.

The significance of Stage 3 NREM becomes evident when considering its role in ensuring that individuals wake up feeling refreshed. This deep stage of sleep is essential for cognitive function, emotional well-being, and physical vitality. Without an adequate amount of Stage 3 NREM, individuals may experience daytime fatigue, difficulty concentrating, and a general sense of lethargy.

Stage 4 REM (Dreaming)

Stage 4 REM, also known as the dreaming stage, is a fascinating and critical phase in the sleep cycle that typically commences approximately 90 minutes after the onset of sleep. This stage is characterized by vivid dreaming and, at times, the occurrence of nightmares. As the body enters this phase, a distinctive set of physiological changes takes place.

One prominent feature of Stage 4 REM is the rapid movement of the eyes from side to side behind closed eyelids. This phenomenon, commonly known as rapid eye movement or REM, is accompanied by an increase in heart rate and breathing. Intriguingly, despite the heightened brain activity resembling that of wakefulness, the muscles of the arms and legs undergo a temporary paralysis. This physiological response serves as a protective mechanism, preventing individuals from physically acting out the scenarios playing out in their dreams.

The duration of each REM cycle can vary, lasting anywhere from 10 minutes to a full hour. Throughout the night, individuals undergo multiple cycles of REM sleep, each contributing to the overall quality of sleep. It is estimated that approximately 25% of total sleep time is spent in REM sleep.

Experts posit that a balanced combination of both REM and non-REM sleep is essential for memory consolidation. During REM sleep, the brain is believed to engage in the process of organizing and storing memories, a crucial function for cognitive well-being. The intricate dance between these different sleep stages contributes to the overall restoration and maintenance of physical and mental health.

Understanding the intricacies of Stage 4 REM sheds light on the multifaceted nature of the sleep cycle. It highlights the orchestrated interplay between physiological changes and cognitive processes, underscoring the importance of a good night's sleep for overall well-being. As we delve into the mysteries of the dreaming stage, we gain valuable insights into the complex and still not entirely understood realm of sleep and its impact on our daily lives.

How much sleep do we need?

The Centers for Disease Control and Prevention
(CDC) has determined that the amount of sleep
required by individuals is contingent upon their age.
As individuals age, they tend to require fewer hours of
sleep in order to remain functional:

- Newborns (0–3 months): 14–17 hours
- Infants (4–12 months): 12–16 hours
- Toddler (1–2 years): 11–14 hours
- Preschool (3–5 years): 10–13 hours
- School age (6–12 years): 9–12 hours
- Teen (13–18 years): 8–10 hours
- Adult (18–60 years): 7-plus hours
- Adult (61–64 years): 7–9 hours
- Adult (65+ years): 7–8 hours

The Biology of Sleep

Circadian Rhythms

Circadian rhythms are intricate, intrinsic biological cycles that play a fundamental role in regulating various physiological and behavioral processes within living organisms. Derived from the Latin words "circa" (meaning "around") and "diem" (meaning "day"), circadian rhythms essentially revolve around a roughly 24-hour day-night cycle. The sleep-wake cycle is one of the most significant and recognized circadian rhythms.

The circadian rhythm is regulated by different parts of the body and is in sync with a circadian rhythm in the brain. This internal clock is directly influenced by environmental cues, especially light, which is why circadian rhythms are tied to the cycle of day and

night.

When properly aligned, a circadian rhythm can promote consistent and restorative sleep. When this circadian rhythm is disrupted, it can lead to serious sleep issues, including insomnia. Research is also revealing that circadian rhythms play an integral role in diverse aspects of physical and mental health.

Neural Mechanisms

The intricate relationship between neural mechanisms and the biological phenomenon of sleep underscores a captivating interplay within the intricate landscape of the human brain. Sleep, a fundamental physiological process, is governed by a complex network of neural circuits and biochemical pathways that orchestrate the transitions between different sleep stages.

At the core of these neural mechanisms is the intricate dance between neurotransmitters, hormones, and various brain regions. The neurotransmitter serotonin, for instance, plays a pivotal role in regulating the sleep-wake cycle, influencing the onset and duration of sleep. Conversely, the neurotransmitter dopamine, associated with wakefulness, acts in opposition to promote alertness.

One of the key brain structures involved in the regulation of sleep is the hypothalamus. Within the hypothalamus lies the suprachiasmatic nucleus (SCN), often referred to as the body's internal clock. The SCN receives input from light-sensitive cells in the retina, helping to synchronize the circadian rhythm with the external day-night cycle. This synchronization is crucial for maintaining a consistent sleep-wake pattern.

The intricate neural mechanisms involved in sleep extend beyond the hypothalamus to encompass the thalamus and various cortical regions. During non-REM (rapid eye movement) sleep, the thalamus plays a role in reducing the flow of sensory information to the cortex, contributing to the characteristic decreased responsiveness to external stimuli. In contrast, REM sleep is associated with heightened cortical activity and vivid dreaming.

Neural oscillations, patterns of synchronized activity among groups of neurons, also play a crucial role in the regulation of sleep stages. Delta waves, for example, dominate the EEG (electroencephalogram) during deep sleep, while theta and alpha waves are more prominent during lighter stages of sleep.

Moreover, the involvement of the amygdala and hippocampus in the processing of emotional and memory-related information during sleep adds another layer of complexity to the neural mechanisms governing this fundamental process. Sleep is now recognized as a crucial period for memory consolidation, where experiences and information acquired during wakefulness are integrated and stored.

Hormonal Regulation

What are hormones? Hormones are chemicals that your body releases into your bloodstream. They're responsible for a bunch of different things in your body, like growth, sex, stress response, and how food you eat turns into energy. All the glands that release hormones are part of the endocrine system.

The intricate process of sleep involves a complex interplay of various physiological mechanisms, with hormonal regulation playing a pivotal role in orchestrating this fundamental aspect of human biology. The intricate dance of hormones orchestrates the different stages of sleep, ensuring a finely tuned balance that is essential for overall well-being.

One key player in the biology of sleep is melatonin, often referred to as the "sleep hormone." Melatonin is produced by the pineal gland in response to diminishing light levels, particularly in the evening. As daylight wanes, the pineal gland releases melatonin into the bloodstream, signaling to the body that it is time to wind down and prepare for sleep. This hormone, therefore, acts as a biological timekeeper, helping to regulate the circadian rhythm—the internal body clock that governs the sleep-wake cycle.

The circadian rhythm is intricately connected to another crucial hormone, cortisol. Often known as the "stress hormone," cortisol follows a diurnal pattern, with levels typically peaking in the early morning to help kickstart the day and gradually decreasing as the day progresses. This cyclical cortisol release complements the circadian rhythm, promoting alertness during waking hours and contributing to the winding down process as bedtime approaches.

Sleep Deprivation

What is sleep deprivation

Sleep deprivation is a condition in which a person does not receive adequate amounts of sleep. It can be a temporary problem, lasting for one or two nights, or a long-term issue that can last for weeks or months. There are numerous causes for sleep deprivation, some of which are benign, but it is also a sign of certain health issues. Everyone needs sleep, and the amount of sleep needed varies depending on age. Some individuals require more sleep to experience a good night's rest, while others require less sleep. However, these exceptions are rare. If your sleep patterns change, either gradually or suddenly, it is important to consult a healthcare professional.

What causes sleep deprivation?

There are many causes of chronic sleep deprivation, but the most common is an emotional response called a conditioned response. When you think about sleep problems or worry about not sleeping enough, these feelings can affect your normal sleep behavior and prolong the length of sleep loss.

You can also be sleep deprived because you choose not to. For example, you choose not to read books, watch TV, or spend time with friends. Certain life events, like a chronic illness, can also cause sleep deprivation.

People with certain illnesses like colds and tonsillitis can get snored, gagged, and wake up early, which can all mess with a regular sleep schedule. Sleep problems like sleep apnea and limb movement disorder can also make it hard to get enough sleep. Plus, certain health issues like asthma or depression can mess with your sleep-wake cycle. And if you take certain medicines like epilepsy or ADHD, they can mess with your night sleep and cause sleep deprivation. And if you're going through a lot of stress in your life, like changing or losing your job, losing a loved one, or moving, you might experience sleep deprivation for a short time.

Environmental elements, such as extreme temperatures, loud noises, and bright lights, can have a detrimental effect on sleep. Additionally, certain lifestyle habits, such as consuming coffee or smoking before bedtime, can cause the nervous system to become preoccupied with worrying about certain matters rather than preparing for sleep. Parents with newborns may also experience sleep deprivation due to the need to care for them. Furthermore, young children and adolescents may suffer from sleep deprivation due to their study-related obligations, such as examinations and assignments. Finally, those over the age of 65 may find it difficult to fall asleep at night due to the aging process and age-related medical conditions.

Symptoms of Sleep Deprivation

Signs of sleep deprivation can range from mild to severe, and if you don't get enough shut-eye, it can lead to some serious issues. Here are some of the most common signs of sleep deprivation:

1. Fatigue: Persistent tiredness and lack of energy are hallmark signs of sleep deprivation. Even if you've had some sleep, the quality may be poor, leading to feelings of exhaustion.

2. Irritability: Sleep-deprived individuals often find themselves more easily agitated, frustrated, or irritable. Emotional resilience tends to be lower when sleep is inadequate.

3. Difficulty Concentrating: Reduced attention span, difficulty focusing, and impaired cognitive

performance are common cognitive symptoms of sleep deprivation. This can impact work, school, and daily activities.

4. Memory Issues: Sleep plays a crucial role in memory consolidation. Sleep-deprived individuals may experience difficulties with short-term and long-term memory.

5. Impaired Judgment: Lack of sleep can affect decision-making abilities and increase the likelihood of poor judgment. This can have serious consequences in activities such as driving.

6. Weakened Immune System: Chronic sleep deprivation can compromise the immune system, making individuals more susceptible to illness and infections.

7. Increased Appetite: Sleep deprivation can disrupt the balance of hormones that regulate appetite, leading to an increase in hunger and a preference for high-calorie foods.

8. Mood Swings: Changes in mood, including heightened emotional responses, increased stress, and a

tendency to react more negatively to situations, are common when sleep is insufficient.

9. Impaired Motor Skills: Coordination and reaction times may be negatively impacted by sleep deprivation, increasing the risk of accidents and injuries.

10. Hallucinations: In extreme cases, prolonged sleep deprivation can lead to hallucinations, both auditory and visual.

It's important to note that the severity of symptoms can vary from person to person, and acute sleep deprivation can often be reversed by getting adequate rest. However, chronic sleep deprivation can have serious health implications and may require intervention. If you consistently experience symptoms of sleep deprivation, it's advisable to consult with a healthcare professional for guidance.

Sleep Effect on Heart

It's clear that if you don't get enough sleep, it can have a negative impact on your heart health. Sleep is a key part of your body's recovery process, and it's important to get enough of it. During the NREM sleep stages, your heart rate slows down, your blood pressure goes down, and your breathing calms down. This helps your heart recover from the strain it's under during the day. Unfortunately, if you're not getting enough sleep, you won't get the benefit of the NREM sleep that helps your heart. This can also be true for people whose sleep is often disturbed. Chronic sleep deprivation can lead to a range of heart problems, like high blood pressure, cholesterol levels, heart attack, being overweight, having diabetes, and having a stroke.

Sleep and Blood Pressure

During a good night's sleep, your blood pressure usually goes down by 10-20%, which is called nocturnal dipping. But if you don't get enough sleep, or if you have sleep problems, your blood pressure won't go down. Studies have shown that elevated blood pressure during the night is linked to high blood pressure in general, and that night blood pressure is even more likely to cause heart problems than day high blood pressure. Not getting enough sleep can lead to stroke and heart attack, as well as kidney problems and less blood to the brain.

Lots of studies have found that sleep deprivation can lead to an increase in your blood pressure during the day. But it doesn't just affect people who don't get enough sleep - it can also affect people who are middle-aged, working long hours in stressful jobs, and have other health issues that could lead to high blood pressure. So, if you're not getting enough sleep, it's likely that your blood pressure will go up.

Sleep and Heart Attacks

If you don't get enough sleep, you're more likely to have a heart attack. It's a type of heart attack that happens when the blood to the heart is blocked, and it can be fatal. Not getting enough sleep can also increase your risk of having a heart attack. A study found that people who slept less than six hours a night were 20% more likely to have one. The NREM sleep cycle helps your heart slow down and recuperate, but REM sleep involves more stress and activity, which can disrupt the balance of the sleep cycle and increase your risk of heart attack. Plus, frequent sleep interruptions can cause stress in your heart, which can lead to a heart attack.

Sleep and Stroke

When blood isn't flowing to the brain, it can cause brain cells to die because they don't have enough oxygen. Ischaemic strokes happen when a clot or plaque gets stuck in an artery. A TIA, or mini-stroke, is just a temporary blockage. Studies have shown that not sleeping enough can make you more likely to have a stroke. Not sleeping raises your blood pressure, which is the main risk factor for stroke. Plus, not sleeping can make it easier for plaque to build up in your arteries, which can lead to mini-strokes.

Sleep and Obesity

Having a high BMI or being overweight or obese is linked to a lot of health issues, like high blood pressure, diabetes, and high cholesterol. It can also lead to heart disease, stroke, and heart attack. Lack of sleep is also linked to obesity, since people who don't get enough sleep (say, seven hours a night) are more likely to be overweight or obese. Sleep helps control the hormones that make us hungry, so when we don't get enough, it can lead to overeating and the urge to eat more high-calorie food.

Sleep and Coronary Heart Disease

Heart disease is a leading cause of death in the United States. It's caused by plaque buildup in the arteries, which makes them hard and narrow. This means the heart can't get enough oxygen and blood. Research has shown that sleep deprivation can lead to atherosclerosis, which is caused by inflammation. The immune system produces white blood cells that collect in the arteries, and if you don't get enough sleep, they can cause inflammation and harden the arteries. Hypertension can also make the arteries less efficient at getting blood to the heart, which can lead to heart disease.

Sleep and Type 2 Diabetes

Diabetes is a long-term condition where your blood sugar gets too high because your body can't process it properly. Too much sugar can damage your blood vessels, which can have a negative impact on your heart health. People with type 2 diabetes are more likely to have heart disease or a stroke than those without it. There are lots of things that can affect your blood sugar, but sleep deprivation can be one of them. Studies have shown that sleep deprivation can make glucose metabolism worse. Poor sleep is linked to prediabetes, which is when your glucose levels are too high and you don't have diabetes. If you've already been diagnosed with diabetes, it can be harder for you to control your blood sugar if you're not getting enough or restless sleep. Poor sleep can also make your arteries harder to harden.

Sleep and Heart Rate

When you're sleeping, your heart rate usually goes down during the NREM stages and then back up when you wake up. But if you're not getting enough sleep, like if you wake up suddenly, it can cause your heart rate to go up. People with sleeping issues are also more likely to complain about having an irregular heartbeat, so it's possible that lack of sleep could be connected to heart palps. A study in older adults also found that people who had a lot of nightmares were more likely to have an irregular heartbeat. If you're having a bad dream, your heart rate can go up, and you might wake up feeling like your heart is racing.

Sleep and Chest Pain

Chest pain can be caused by a variety of things, like angina pectoris, which is when your heart beats too fast and your blood pressure gets too high. Studies have shown that sleep deprivation can also cause chest pain. Not only that, but if you have heartburn or acid reflux, you're more likely to experience chest pain. Plus, if you have unexplained chest pain, it's more likely to be linked to insomnia. We don't know exactly how stress and anxiety can cause chest pain, but it could be related to panic reactions, which are more common when you're not getting enough sleep.

Sleep and Heart Health During Pregnancy

Pregnancy puts a lot of pressure on your heart, and some women experience heart issues during their pregnancy. For instance, high blood pressure can start or get worse during pregnancy, which can be dangerous for both you and your baby. A lot of pregnant women also experience sleep problems, like insomnia and sleep apnea, which have been linked to a higher risk of heart problems later in life. Researchers are trying to figure out how to get better sleep during pregnancy, which could also help reduce high blood pressure and other heart problems.

Sleep for People With Heart Disease

It is essential for individuals with cardiovascular disorders to prioritize sleep, as sleep deprivation can have a detrimental effect on the heart. In fact, research has indicated that improved sleep may reduce the risk of heart attacks and other cardiovascular issues in individuals who are already at high risk. However, certain heart conditions can impede sleep, such as diabetes, which can lead to frequent nighttime urination. Additionally, other cardiovascular disorders can cause chest discomfort when attempting to sleep. Furthermore, worry and stress related to heart health can make it difficult to relax and fall asleep. Therefore, it is beneficial to discuss heart-healthy sleep with a doctor, who can provide a tailored plan to improve sleep while also focusing on other lifestyle factors that are beneficial for the heart and overall health.

Sleep Tips for People With Heart Problems

While there is no one-size-fits-all solution, specific suggestions can often assist individuals with heart issues in achieving better sleep.

- Establish relaxation strategies: If heart-related concerns trigger anxiety, they may keep your mind active when you are trying to unwind for sleep. Techniques such as deep breathing, yoga, gentle stretching, and mindfulness meditation are beneficial approaches for those grappling with sleep issues related to pericarditis (inflammation around the heart), heart disease, or other cardiac problems causing chest pain.

- Maintain a consistent sleep schedule: Adhering to the same bedtime and wake-up time every day is widely recognized as a crucial method for promoting consistent and healthy sleep each night.

- Create a conducive bedroom environment: Tailor your sleep space to meet your needs by ensuring it features a comfortable mattress and pillow, maintains a pleasant temperature, and maximizes quietness and darkness.

- Avoid sleep-disrupting factors: Both alcohol and caffeine can impede sleep and are best avoided at night. Excessive use of electronic devices, including your cell phone, can also disrupt sleep patterns. Experts recommend refraining from using these devices for at least an hour before bedtime.

Does Sleeping Position Affect Heart Health?

Limited evidence exists linking an individual's sleep position to their overall heart health. Some studies, particularly those focusing on individuals with congestive heart failure, suggest that sleeping on the left side may induce changes in heart and lung function. Congestive heart failure occurs when there is an accumulation of fluid in the lungs or other parts of the body due to ineffective blood pumping by the heart. Research indicates that individuals with congestive heart failure often avoid sleeping on their left side, with a more pronounced effect observed in those with larger heart dimensions. The exact reason for this avoidance is unknown, but it may be connected to how this sleeping position alters the heart's positioning, exerts pressure on the lungs, or affects the feeling of a beating heart against the chest wall.

It is essential to note that while studies reveal a tendency for people with heart failure to avoid left-side sleeping, there is no evidence proving that this sleeping position causes heart problems. According to current research, an individual's sleep position is not considered a risk factor for heart disease or other cardiovascular issues.

Sleep in depression

Sleep patterns in individuals experiencing depression are characterized by brief, shallow, and fragmented episodes, featuring rapid eye movement (REM) during the early phases of sleep and heightened eye movement. This phenomenon is particularly prevalent in those with unipolar depression (depression without manic episodes) and older individuals displaying increased agitation. In contrast, bipolar disorder tends to manifest differently, often presenting with excessive sleepiness. To gain insight into the sleep quality of those with major depressive disorder, it's essential to consider the following: the time span between sleep onset and the initiation of the first REM period is typically shorter in depressed individuals. In non-depressed individuals, the initial REM period is relatively brief and extends as the night progresses. However, depressed individuals exhibit a prolonged initial REM period that doesn't increase in duration throughout the night.

During this initial REM period, there is a significant increase in the number of eye movements per minute (REM density). Initially, it was thought that this short REM latency could serve as a biological indicator of depression, aiding psychiatrists in understanding the physiology of the condition. Yet, subsequent research revealed that a short REM latency is not specific to depression and can occur in various conditions, making it a sensitive but not highly specific biomarker for depression. This phenomenon, coupled with a decrease in slow-wave sleep patterns, contributes to our understanding of sleep regulation models.

Modifying one's sleep patterns can be an effective approach to treating depression. Studies indicate that altering sleep, such as eliminating REM sleep, experiencing one night of total sleep, or staying awake for an extended period, can effectively reduce depression symptoms comparable to the impact of antidepressants. Unfortunately, these methods require substantial effort, making them less practical. However, the crucial takeaway is that since changing sleep can influence the course of depression, poor sleep is not just a consequence of depression; it's likely a contributing factor to the mood disorder's development. Post-Traumatic Stress Disorder (PTSD) arises from exposure to highly stressful, frightening, or distressing events. Approximately half of individuals with PTSD experience nightmares, and for some, the difficulty in achieving restful sleep becomes so pronounced that they develop a fear of going to bed.

Individuals experiencing PTSD often exhibit an elevated Rapid Eye Movement (REM) density, indicating an increased frequency of eye movements during REM sleep. This augmentation is particularly prevalent among those reliving the traumatic experience and grappling with heightened anxiety. Concurrently, individuals with PTSD commonly encounter additional sleep-related challenges, such as a high prevalence of sleep-disorder breathing in over half of the affected population, and excessive leg movements in 35-77 percent of cases.

The correlation between sleep patterns and PTSD remains somewhat elusive. Certain studies suggest that individuals grappling with significant sleep disturbances within the initial weeks following a traumatic event, such as a car crash, are more prone to developing PTSD within the subsequent six to twelve months. Interestingly, it's plausible that pre-existing sleep issues might serve as a protective factor against the onset of PTSD in the future.

Considering the role of sleep in the consolidation of long-term memory, it follows that the absence of proper sleep immediately after a traumatic incident may diminish the likelihood of the trauma persisting emotionally over an extended period. Treatment for sleep-related problems in PTSD pursues at least two primary objectives. One objective involves addressing concurrent sleep disorders; for instance, effective treatment of sleep-disorder breathing often correlates with a reduction in PTSD symptoms. Prazosin, a medication that blocks certain norepinephrine receptors, is frequently prescribed by doctors to enhance sleep quality and overall clinical well-being. It may also alleviate nightmares, albeit without official approval for this purpose.

However, the use of prazosin is subject to restrictions, such as avoiding excessive lowering of blood pressure. Given that many individuals with PTSD also exhibit symptoms of depression or anxiety, appropriate medications like Selective Serotonin Reuptake Inhibitors (SSRIs) including sertraline and paroxetine are commonly employed. Additionally, psychotherapeutic interventions, such as imagery rehearsal, retraining, and cognitive-behavioral therapy, can prove beneficial in managing certain symptoms. Even with the necessary assistance, it's not uncommon for individuals to continue experiencing sleep-related issues in the long term.

Sleep and Memory

Memory Consolidation

Memory consolidation is the process of making a memory last as long as possible. Proper memory function requires each of these phases; however, acquisition and recall occur only when awake while memory consolidation occurs during sleep by strengthening the brain connections that produce memories.

Researchers believe that unique brainwave properties throughout different phases of sleep are linked to memory development. Consolidation is a way of making a memory stick to existing knowledge networks by holding it steady on the memory trace, which can be a lot of memory waves of short and long-term consolidation processes.

The role of sleep in memory consolidation is a fascinating aspect of cognitive function, shedding light on the intricate relationship between our nightly slumber and the way our brains organize and store information. Memory consolidation refers to the process by which newly acquired information is stabilized, strengthened, and integrated into existing memory networks, promoting long-term retention.

During sleep, especially in the deeper stages such as slow-wave sleep (SWS) and rapid eye movement (REM) sleep, the brain undergoes a series of complex physiological and neurochemical changes that actively contribute to memory consolidation. One key player in this process is the hippocampus, a region of the brain critical for the formation of new memories.

Firstly, during slow-wave sleep, the brain engages in a rhythmic pattern of electrical activity known as sharp-wave ripples. These events are believed to facilitate the transfer of information from the hippocampus to the neocortex, the outer layer of the brain responsible for higher cognitive functions. This transfer is crucial for the transformation of fragile, short-term memories into more robust, long-term memories.

Secondly, REM sleep, characterized by vivid dreaming and rapid eye movements, is implicated in the consolidation of emotional and procedural memories. It is during REM sleep that the brain selectively strengthens and consolidates memories with emotional content, providing a subjective richness to our recollections.

Furthermore, sleep is associated with changes in the levels of neurotransmitters, such as acetylcholine and serotonin, which play essential roles in memory processing. The interplay of these neurotransmitters during different sleep stages contributes to the optimization of synaptic connections, enhancing the efficiency of memory storage.

Interestingly, research suggests that the benefits of sleep on memory consolidation are not uniform across all types of memories. While declarative memories (facts and events) tend to benefit from the consolidation processes during slow-wave sleep, procedural memories (skills and habits) may be more effectively consolidated during REM sleep.

Sleep serves as a critical and dynamic period for memory consolidation. The orchestrated interplay of different sleep stages, neural processes, and neurotransmitter activity creates an environment conducive to the transformation of recent experiences into lasting memories. Recognizing the significance of a good night's sleep not only for overall well-being but also for the enhancement of cognitive functions underscores the importance of prioritizing healthy sleep habits in our daily lives.

Dreaming and Memory Processing

Dreaming and memory processing are intricate facets of the human brain's complex functions. When we delve into the realm of dreaming, we step into a mysterious landscape where the mind weaves narratives that often defy the laws of logic and physics. Despite the surreal and fantastical nature of dreams, they play a vital role in the consolidation and processing of memories.

During the various stages of sleep, the brain undergoes a sophisticated dance of neuronal activity. One prominent feature of this dance is the rapid eye movement (REM) stage, where dreams are most vivid and memorable. It is within this stage that the brain appears to sift through the vast array of experiences and information gathered during waking hours, selecting, consolidating, and even discarding elements.

Dreams seem to serve as a theater for the mind to replay and reinterpret daily experiences. In doing so, the brain is thought to strengthen memories, transferring them from short-term storage to more stable long-term storage. This process, known as memory consolidation, is crucial for learning and adapting to the challenges of the waking world.

The content of dreams often reflects the emotional tone of our experiences, highlighting events that triggered strong feelings. This emotional salience may act as a guiding force for the brain, prioritizing certain memories over others. Dreams, in this sense, become a narrative tool through which the mind prioritizes, organizes, and integrates memories into the vast tapestry of one's cognitive landscape.

Moreover, dreaming is not a uniform experience; it is a diverse spectrum of mental activities that can range from the mundane to the surreal. Some dreams may vividly replay recent events, while others may transport us to fantastical realms constructed from the amalgamation of our thoughts, fears, and desires. This diversity in dream content suggests a dynamic and flexible memory processing system that adapts to the unique needs and challenges of each individual.

Beyond memory consolidation, dreams may also contribute to problem-solving and creative thinking. The unbridled nature of dreaming allows the mind to make novel connections between seemingly unrelated concepts, fostering creativity and innovation. Artists, writers, and scientists throughout history have attested to the inspirational power of dreams in generating new ideas and insights.

While the precise mechanisms linking dreaming and memory processing are not fully understood, research continues to shed light on the intricate relationship between these cognitive phenomena. As technology advances, tools such as functional magnetic resonance imaging (fMRI) and electroencephalography (EEG) provide glimpses into the neural ballet that unfolds during sleep, offering clues about the role dreams play in shaping our memories and, by extension, our understanding of the world. In unraveling the enigma of dreaming and memory, we unravel the intricate workings of the mind itself, a journey that continues to captivate scientists and dreamers alike.

Sleep and Physical Health

Immune System Function

The immune system is a complex and highly orchestrated network of cells, tissues, and organs that work together to defend the body against harmful invaders, such as bacteria, viruses, fungi, and other pathogens. Its primary function is to distinguish between the body's own cells and foreign substances, and then mount a targeted response to eliminate or neutralize anything that poses a threat to health.

One of the key components of the immune system is white blood cells, which come in various types, each playing a unique role in the defense mechanism. Phagocytes, for instance, are like the body's scavengers, engulfing and digesting foreign particles. T cells are specialized cells that recognize and destroy infected or abnormal cells directly. B cells produce antibodies, proteins that can bind to specific pathogens and neutralize them or mark them for destruction.

The immune system operates in two main ways: the innate immune response and the adaptive immune response. The innate response is the body's immediate, non-specific defense against a wide range of pathogens. This includes physical barriers like the skin, as well as cellular and molecular components that are always ready to respond quickly to infections.

On the other hand, the adaptive immune response is highly specific and involves the recognition of specific antigens (molecules on the surface of pathogens) by T and B cells. Once the immune system encounters a new pathogen, it "learns" from the experience and develops memory cells. This immunological memory allows the immune system to mount a faster and more robust response upon subsequent exposures to the same pathogen, providing the basis for vaccines and long-lasting immunity.

The immune system also plays a crucial role in maintaining overall health by recognizing and removing damaged or abnormal cells, such as cancer cells. It operates not only in the bloodstream but also in lymphoid tissues, such as the spleen and lymph nodes, which serve as command centers for immune cell communication and activation.

Balancing act is vital for the immune system – it needs to be robust enough to defend against pathogens but also regulated to prevent excessive reactions that can lead to autoimmune diseases, where the immune system mistakenly attacks the body's own cells.

The immune system is a dynamic and sophisticated defense mechanism that safeguards the body against a myriad of threats. Its ability to discriminate between self and non-self, remember past encounters, and mount tailored responses is essential for maintaining health and well-being.

Cellular Repair and Growth

During the restorative phase of sleep, the human body undergoes a remarkable process of cellular repair and growth, contributing significantly to overall health and well-being. This intricate physiological dance occurs predominantly during the deeper stages of sleep, particularly in the slow-wave and REM (Rapid Eye Movement) phases.

One key player in this nocturnal rejuvenation is the release of growth hormone. This hormone, secreted by the pituitary gland, plays a pivotal role in stimulating growth, cell reproduction, and regeneration. Throughout the night, growth hormone levels surge, promoting the repair of tissues and muscles that may have experienced wear and tear during daily activities.

Moreover, the body engages in a process known as cellular autophagy. This mechanism involves the removal of damaged or malfunctioning cellular components. Think of it as a cellular recycling program, where the body breaks down and eliminates old, worn-out structures, making room for the creation of new, healthier cells. This not only aids in tissue repair but also helps in maintaining the integrity and functionality of various organs.

The brain, too, takes advantage of the downtime during sleep to consolidate memories and clear out metabolic byproducts that accumulate throughout the day. The glymphatic system, a waste clearance system in the brain, becomes more active during sleep, flushing out toxins and debris that could contribute to neurological disorders if allowed to build up.

Additionally, the immune system gets a boost during sleep. Various immune functions, such as the production of immune cells and antibodies, are heightened, enhancing the body's ability to defend against infections and illnesses. This is crucial for maintaining overall health and resilience against pathogens.

In summary, sleep serves as a critical period for the body to repair, regenerate, and grow at the cellular level. The orchestrated release of hormones, the elimination of cellular waste, and the fortification of the immune system collectively contribute to the overall maintenance and optimization of bodily functions. Recognizing the importance of quality sleep underscores the significance of adopting healthy sleep habits for sustained well-being.

Impact on Cardiovascular Health

Sleep plays a crucial role in maintaining optimal cardiovascular health, and its impact on the cardiovascular system is profound and multifaceted.

If you don't get enough or even good sleep, you could be at risk for a bunch of different heart problems. High blood pressure is one of them, and it can be caused by not getting enough sleep. When you're sleeping, your body goes through different stages that help keep your blood pressure in check. But if you're not getting enough sleep or your sleep cycles are irregular, it can lead to your blood pressure getting higher and higher over time.

Furthermore, insufficient sleep has been associated with an increased risk of atherosclerosis, a condition characterized by the accumulation of plaque in the arteries. The inflammatory response and stress hormones that can be triggered by lack of sleep contribute to the development of arterial plaque, potentially compromising blood flow and increasing the risk of cardiovascular events such as heart attacks and strokes.

Sleep also plays a vital role in regulating glucose metabolism and insulin sensitivity. Disruptions in sleep patterns, such as those seen in conditions like sleep apnea, can lead to insulin resistance and an increased risk of type 2 diabetes. Diabetes, in turn, is a significant risk factor for cardiovascular disease, creating a complex interplay between sleep, metabolic health, and cardiovascular well-being.

Moreover, the autonomic nervous system, which regulates heart rate and blood vessel function, experiences significant fluctuations during different sleep stages. This delicate balance can be disturbed when sleep is compromised, potentially leading to irregular heart rhythms (arrhythmias) and an increased workload on the heart.

On a positive note, obtaining sufficient and high-quality sleep has been associated with a lower risk of cardiovascular events. Adequate sleep supports overall cardiovascular function by allowing the heart and blood vessels to rest and recover. It promotes a healthy balance of hormones and reduces stress on the cardiovascular system, contributing to better heart health.

Therefore, the impact of sleep on cardiovascular health is intricate and substantial. Consistent, good-quality sleep is essential for maintaining optimal blood pressure, preventing the development of atherosclerosis, regulating metabolism, and promoting overall cardiovascular well-being. Prioritizing healthy sleep habits is, therefore, a crucial component of a comprehensive approach to cardiovascular health.

Emotional Regulation During Sleep

Dreams and Emotional Processing

Dreams are enigmatic phenomena that unfold within the realm of sleep, serving as a mysterious tapestry woven from the threads of our subconscious. Amidst the tranquil landscapes of slumber, the mind embarks on a captivating journey, navigating through the intricate corridors of emotions and memories. At the heart of this nocturnal odyssey lies the profound process of emotional integration and understanding, a phenomenon that has intrigued scholars, psychologists, and dream enthusiasts alike.

As the night unfolds its velvet curtain, dreams emerge as the subconscious mind's canvas, painting vivid scenes that often mirror our deepest fears, desires, and unresolved conflicts. It is within this surreal theater of the mind that emotions take center stage, dancing with unrestrained fervor and weaving a narrative that may be both fantastical and deeply personal.

One of the key roles dreams play is in emotional processing, a nocturnal therapy where the mind confronts, revisits, and attempts to reconcile unresolved feelings. The symbolism in dreams acts as a symbolic language, expressing sentiments that may be too complex or buried within the recesses of waking consciousness. Emotions, both raw and nuanced, find expression in the form of surreal landscapes, symbolic interactionism, and abstract scenarios.

During sleep, the brain engages in a unique choreography, orchestrating the processing of emotional experiences from the day. This intricate dance involves the integration of new memories, the consolidation of learned information, and the emotional regulation essential for mental well-being. Dreams, in this context, become the narrative thread that binds together the disparate elements of our emotional landscape.

Moreover, dreams may serve as a form of rehearsal for real-life situations, allowing the mind to explore various emotional responses in a safe and controlled environment. This rehearsal can contribute to emotional resilience, providing an opportunity for the subconscious to experiment with different scenarios and emotional outcomes.

The relationship between dreams and emotional processing is a dynamic interplay, with each influencing the other in a nuanced ballet. Emotional experiences during waking hours shape the content of dreams, while the emotional intensity within dreams can influence waking emotions. This bidirectional flow underscores the intricate connection between the conscious and subconscious realms of the mind.

Sleep and Mental Health

Sleep plays a pivotal role in maintaining optimal mental health, serving as a cornerstone for cognitive function, emotional well-being, and overall psychological resilience. The intricate interplay between sleep and mental health is a dynamic relationship, with each influencing and shaping the other in profound ways.

One of the primary functions of sleep is the consolidation of memories and the enhancement of learning processes. During the various stages of sleep, particularly the restorative deep sleep known as slow-wave sleep (SWS), the brain engages in memory consolidation, helping to solidify and organize information acquired throughout the day. This process is crucial for cognitive functions such as problem-solving, decision-making, and creativity, all of which are integral components of mental health.

Furthermore, sleep plays a vital role in regulating mood and emotional well-being. Sleep deprivation has been linked to heightened emotional reactivity, increased irritability, and a decreased ability to cope with stress. Adequate sleep fosters emotional resilience, allowing individuals to navigate life's challenges with a greater sense of equilibrium. Disruptions in sleep patterns, whether due to insomnia, sleep apnea, or other sleep disorders, can contribute to mood disorders such as depression and anxiety.

The impact of sleep on mental health is bidirectional. Mental health conditions, such as anxiety and depression, can, in turn, disrupt normal sleep patterns, creating a cycle that exacerbates both the mental health issue and the sleep disturbance. This reciprocal relationship underscores the importance of addressing sleep as a fundamental component of mental health care.

The regulation of neurotransmitters, including serotonin and dopamine, is intricately connected to both sleep and mental health. Sleep disturbances can disrupt the delicate balance of these neurotransmitters, contributing to mood disorders. Conversely, mental health conditions can influence sleep by altering the release and reception of neurotransmitters, leading to difficulties falling asleep or staying asleep.

In the realm of psychiatric disorders, conditions like bipolar disorder and schizophrenia often exhibit disturbances in sleep patterns. The circadian rhythm, the body's internal clock regulating sleep-wake cycles, is frequently disrupted in these disorders, underscoring the intricate link between sleep and mental health.

Developing and maintaining healthy sleep habits, often referred to as sleep hygiene, is a crucial aspect of promoting mental well-being. Consistent sleep schedules, creating a comfortable sleep environment, and adopting relaxation techniques before bedtime are essential practices for ensuring restorative sleep.

Recognizing the symbiotic relationship between sleep and mental health highlights the importance of a holistic approach to well-being. Mental health interventions should not only address psychological and emotional aspects but also incorporate strategies to promote healthy sleep. As researchers delve deeper into the complex connections between sleep and mental health, a comprehensive understanding emerges, emphasizing the significance of fostering a healthy sleep environment for the promotion and preservation of mental well-being.

Evolutionary Perspectives on Sleep

Adaptive Significance

The adaptive significance of evolutionary perspectives on sleep delves into the profound biological and ecological reasons behind the evolution of sleep as a ubiquitous and essential phenomenon across the animal kingdom. Evolutionary theories posit that the characteristics of sleep have evolved over time, driven by selective pressures that confer survival and reproductive advantages to species.

One prominent perspective revolves around the concept of energy conservation. Sleep is seen as a mechanism to reduce metabolic demands during periods of inactivity, allowing organisms to allocate energy more efficiently. This adaptation is particularly crucial for species with high metabolic rates, as sleep aids in maintaining an optimal balance between energy expenditure and conservation.

Another vital aspect of the adaptive significance of sleep lies in its role in memory consolidation and cognitive function. Sleep, especially the rapid eye movement (REM) and slow-wave sleep (SWS) stages, is implicated in enhancing learning, memory retention, and problem-solving skills. This suggests that the evolution of sleep is intricately linked to cognitive processes, providing an adaptive advantage to species that can effectively integrate and utilize information gathered during waking hours.

Furthermore, sleep serves as a critical component of predator-prey dynamics and overall safety. Nocturnal sleep patterns, for instance, might have evolved as a strategy for prey animals to avoid predators during their most active periods. On the flip side, predators may have developed adaptations that allow them to be more effective during low-light conditions, thereby increasing their chances of successful hunts.

Social factors also play a role in the adaptive significance of sleep. Group-living species, in particular, may synchronize their sleep-wake cycles to enhance coordination and communication within the group. This social synchronization can improve the efficiency of activities such as foraging, protection, and reproductive behaviors.

Additionally, the immune system's function is intricately tied to sleep. Evolutionary perspectives suggest that sleep facilitates immune responses, aiding in the body's ability to combat infections and diseases. This highlights the adaptive advantage of a well-regulated sleep cycle in maintaining overall health and increasing the likelihood of reproductive success.

Sleep Patterns Across Species

Sleep patterns vary widely across different species, showcasing the intricate and diverse ways in which organisms rest and rejuvenate. From mammals to birds, reptiles to insects, each group has developed unique adaptations to meet their specific physiological and ecological needs.

Mammals, including humans, often display distinct sleep phases, such as REM (rapid eye movement) and non-REM sleep. These phases are characterized by different brain activities, with REM sleep associated with vivid dreaming. The duration and structure of sleep vary among mammals, influenced by factors like body size, metabolic rate, and environmental factors.

Birds, on the other hand, exhibit unihemispheric slow-wave sleep, a phenomenon where one hemisphere of the brain sleeps while the other remains alert. This adaptation allows certain bird species to rest while maintaining awareness of their surroundings, crucial for survival in potentially dangerous environments.

Reptiles, including snakes and lizards, have more flexible sleep patterns. Some species exhibit unihemispheric sleep, similar to birds, while others engage in prolonged periods of inactivity. The ability to regulate body temperature is a key factor influencing reptilian sleep, with some species adjusting their sleep patterns in response to ambient temperature changes.

Insects, with their highly diverse array of species, also showcase a wide range of sleep patterns. Some insects, like bees, exhibit sleep-like states that are essential for memory consolidation, while others, such as certain butterflies, undergo periods of inactivity during their life cycle.

Marine mammals, like dolphins and whales, present another fascinating dimension to sleep patterns. These animals, being conscious breathers, experience unihemispheric sleep, allowing one hemisphere of the brain to remain active while the other rests. This adaptation enables them to surface for air periodically, ensuring their survival in aquatic environments.

The study of sleep patterns across species not only provides insights into the evolution of sleep but also highlights the intricate interplay between biology, behavior, and environment. Understanding these variations contributes to our appreciation of the diverse strategies organisms have evolved to balance the need for rest with the demands of their ecological niches.

Modern Challenges to Sleep

Technology and Sleep Disruption

In the age of technological advancement, our nights have become battlegrounds between sleep and screens. The proliferation of electronic devices, from smartphones to tablets, has introduced a constant stream of blue light, a disruptor of our circadian rhythm. The very devices designed to connect us often act as silent saboteurs, delaying the release of melatonin and tricking our brains into thinking it's still daytime. The allure of scrolling through social media or binge-watching captivating content creates a digital dance that often lasts well into the late hours, robbing individuals of the restorative sleep they desperately need. The challenge lies not just in the existence of these technologies, but in establishing healthy boundaries to protect the sacred realm of sleep from the invasion of the digital world.

Blue Light Exposure:

One of the primary culprits behind technology-induced sleep disruption is the pervasive use of screens emitting blue light. Devices such as smartphones, tablets, and computers emit a significant amount of blue light, which can interfere with the production of melatonin, a hormone responsible for regulating sleep-wake cycles. Prolonged exposure to blue light, especially during the evening hours, can suppress melatonin production, leading to difficulties falling asleep and disrupted circadian rhythms.

Social Media and FOMO:

The advent of social media platforms has transformed the way we connect with others, but it has also introduced a new dimension to sleep disruption. The fear of missing out (FOMO) driven by social media engagement can keep individuals glued to their screens, even late into the night. Constant notifications, updates, and the compulsion to stay digitally connected contribute to heightened stress levels, making it challenging for individuals to unwind and achieve restful sleep.

The 24/7 Work Culture:

Technology has enabled a 24/7 work culture where individuals can be connected to their jobs at any time. The accessibility of work emails, messages, and collaborative tools can extend working hours beyond the traditional nine-to-five, blurring the boundaries between work and personal life. This constant connectivity can lead to increased stress and anxiety, making it difficult for individuals to detach from work-related concerns when it's time to sleep.

Gaming and Virtual Escapism:

The immersive nature of video games and virtual reality experiences offers a thrilling escape for many, but this comes at the expense of sleep. Gaming sessions often extend late into the night, affecting both the duration and quality of sleep. The adrenaline rush from intense gameplay and the cognitive engagement required can lead to difficulty winding down before bedtime, exacerbating sleep disruption.

Tips for Mitigating Technology-Induced Sleep Disruption:

1. Utilize blue light filters on electronic devices, especially during the evening hours, to minimize the impact on melatonin production.

2. Set specific times to disconnect from electronic devices, especially those emitting blue light, at least an hour before bedtime.

3. Designate the bedroom as a tech-free zone and create a calming environment conducive to sleep.

4. Establish boundaries for social media engagement, particularly during the evening, to reduce the impact of FOMO on sleep.

5. Set clear boundaries between work and personal time to prevent work-related stress from interfering with sleep.

Impact of Work Schedules

In the fast-paced landscape of modern work, traditional nine-to-five schedules have given way to a diverse array of working hours. The 24/7 connectivity brought about by globalization and the advent of remote work has blurred the lines between professional life and personal time. Employees find themselves grappling with irregular shift patterns, night shifts, and the constant pressure to be available around the clock. This irregularity disrupts the body's natural circadian rhythm, leading to a cascade of consequences for sleep health. The struggle to balance professional commitments and the fundamental need for adequate rest creates a dichotomy where individuals are forced to navigate the delicate equilibrium between meeting job expectations and maintaining their well-being. The challenge is not just about restructuring work hours but fostering a culture that prioritizes the importance of sleep in sustaining long-term productivity and overall health. The relationship between work schedules and sleep is complex, with different schedules affecting sleep patterns and overall well-being in diverse ways.

1. Shift Work and Sleep Disruptions:
   Shift work, involving irregular or non-traditional hours, is a common factor that significantly affects sleep. Those working night shifts or rotating shifts often experience disruptions to their circadian rhythm, the body's natural internal clock. This misalignment can lead to difficulties falling asleep, staying asleep, and obtaining the recommended amount of restorative sleep.

2. Long Work Hours and Sleep Deprivation:
   Extended work hours contribute to sleep deprivation, a condition with profound consequences for physical

and mental health. Individuals working long hours may sacrifice sleep to meet job demands, leading to a cumulative sleep debt. Persistent sleep deprivation is associated with increased risks of accidents, impaired cognitive function, and a heightened susceptibility to various health issues.

3. Flexibility and Sleep Quality:

The flexibility of work schedules can either mitigate or exacerbate sleep-related challenges. While flexible schedules may allow individuals to adapt their work hours to their preferred sleep-wake patterns, they can also lead to irregular sleep routines. Maintaining a consistent sleep schedule is crucial for quality sleep, and disruptions to this routine can negatively impact overall sleep quality.

4. Job Stress and Sleep Disturbances:

High levels of job-related stress can contribute to sleep disturbances. Individuals with demanding and stressful jobs may experience difficulty unwinding before bedtime, leading to insomnia or restless sleep. Chronic stress can also contribute to the development of sleep disorders and exacerbate existing sleep-related issues.

5. Technology and Blurred Boundaries:

Modern work environments often involve the use of technology, allowing for remote work and constant connectivity. While this flexibility can enhance work-life balance, it can also blur the boundaries between work and personal life, potentially encroaching on sleep time. The temptation to check emails or complete tasks during non-traditional hours can disrupt sleep patterns.

Sleep Disorders

There are many sleep disorders that can have a negative impact on your heart health. One of the most common is Insomnia, which is often accompanied by poor sleep quality and can lead to increased cardiovascular health risks. Another is Obstructive Sleep Apnea (OSA), a breathing disorder that has been linked to heart disease and obesity, diabetes, and stroke, as well as high blood pressure. Patients with OSA experience lapses in breathing while sleeping, when their airways become blocked. This interrupted breathing from OSA can lead to fragmented sleep, one of the reasons why the condition is associated with multiple cardiovascular problems. Additionally, interrupted respiration can reduce the amount of oxygen available in your blood, which can worsen the effects of OSA on your heart. Disorders of abnormal movement while sleeping, like restless leg syndrome or periodic limb movement disorder (LMD), have also been linked with heart problems. The exact cause of these disorders is unknown, but it may be linked to abnormal activation of your cardiovascular system, which results in elevated and varying heart rates and blood pressure.

Circadian rhythm sleep disorder (CRD) is a sleep disorder that occurs when your circadian rhythm is out of sync with day and night. People with CRD have a higher risk of high blood pressure, obesity, diabetes, and stroke or heart attack.

Insomnia

Sleep disorders are a diverse array of conditions that impede the normal pattern of sleep, affecting the duration and quality of rest individuals experience. One prominent sleep disorder is insomnia, a condition characterized by persistent difficulty in falling asleep, staying asleep, or both. Insomnia can manifest as a short-term issue or become a chronic condition, significantly impacting an individual's overall well-being and daily functioning.

Insomnia is characterized by a lack of ability to fall asleep or remain asleep, resulting in an unrefreshed wakefulness. Complaints of daytime irritability, such as feeling tired or disoriented, may also arise, even if there has been a sufficient amount of sleep during the night.

The most frequent single symptom of insomnia is multiple awakenings throughout the night or lack of restful sleep; however, the majority of individuals with insomnia experience a combination of symptoms, such as difficulty falling asleep and frequent awakenings. The nature of a person's insomnia symptoms may vary over time; some evidence suggests that individuals with one symptom (e.g., difficulty falling asleep) may experience a more fluctuating pattern, whereas those with several symptoms (e.g. difficulty falling asleep and multiple awakenings) may experience more consistent patterns. A lot of people in the US and UK have trouble sleeping at night, and 10% of them say their insomnia affects their day-to-day lives. This includes feeling tired, impulsive, or irritable, having trouble remembering things, and having trouble with relationships. People who have these issues tend to use medical care more, like going to the ER, going to the doctor, and making phone calls. Women are more likely to have sleep problems than men, and it's more common for parents than for those without kids in the home (66% vs. 54%). Most studies show that the number of sleep complaints increases over time, but the highest rate is seen in older people, with 35-64 year olds having the highest rate, and people over 65 having the lowest rate. There's not much of a link between income and insomnia, but the higher the income, the lower the rate.

There are several subtypes of insomnia, each with its unique characteristics. Onset insomnia refers to the difficulty in falling asleep initially, often resulting from factors like stress, anxiety, or environmental disturbances. Maintenance insomnia, on the other hand, involves difficulty staying asleep, leading to frequent awakenings during the night. Individuals with this subtype may find themselves waking up too early and struggling to resume sleep.

The causes of insomnia are multifaceted and can include psychological, physiological, and environmental factors. Stress and anxiety, whether related to work, relationships, or other life events, are common contributors to insomnia. Additionally, medical conditions such as chronic pain, respiratory disorders, or hormonal imbalances can disrupt sleep patterns. Environmental factors like excessive noise, uncomfortable room temperature, or irregular sleep schedules can also exacerbate insomnia.

The consequences of insomnia extend beyond mere fatigue. Persistent lack of sleep can lead to a range of health issues, including impaired cognitive function, mood disturbances such as irritability and depression, weakened immune system, and an increased risk of accidents due to impaired alertness. Moreover, chronic insomnia is often associated with a higher likelihood of developing other medical conditions, such as cardiovascular diseases and metabolic disorders.

Addressing insomnia typically involves a multifaceted approach. Behavioral interventions, such as cognitive-behavioral therapy for insomnia (CBT-I), aim to modify thoughts and behaviors that contribute to sleep difficulties. Lifestyle changes, including adopting a regular sleep schedule, creating a conducive sleep environment, and limiting stimulants like caffeine close to bedtime, are crucial components of insomnia management. In some cases, medications may be prescribed to facilitate sleep, but these are often considered a short-term solution due to potential side effects and the risk of dependence.

Understanding and addressing insomnia require a comprehensive evaluation that considers both the physical and psychological aspects of an individual's well-being. By identifying and addressing the underlying causes, healthcare professionals can develop tailored interventions to help individuals overcome the challenges posed by insomnia and regain restful, rejuvenating sleep.

Sleep Apnea

Sleep Apnea is a sleep disorder where the individual experiences pauses in breathing or shallow breaths while sleeping. There are two main types:

1. Obstructive Sleep Apnea (OSA): The more common type, OSA, occurs when the muscles in the throat relax excessively, causing a temporary blockage of the airway.

2. Central Sleep Apnea (CSA): This type is less common and results from a failure of the brain to transmit the appropriate signals to the muscles that control breathing.

Causes and Risk Factors:
Sleep Apnea can be caused by a variety of factors, including obesity, genetics, age, and underlying health conditions. Risk factors also include a family history of sleep apnea, use of alcohol or sedatives, and smoking.

Symptoms:
The symptoms of Sleep Apnea can be subtle and are often noticed by a bed partner. Common signs include loud snoring, abrupt awakenings accompanied by a choking or gasping sound, and excessive daytime sleepiness. Individuals with Sleep Apnea may also experience difficulty concentrating and irritability.

Health Implications:
Sleep Apnea can cause serious health issues if not addressed. The repeated interruptions in breathing can result in poor oxygenation of the blood, contributing to cardiovascular issues such as high blood pressure, heart attacks, and strokes. Additionally, Sleep Apnea has been linked to diabetes and an increased risk of accidents due to daytime sleepiness.

Diagnosis and Treatment:
Diagnosis often involves a sleep study, where the individual's sleep patterns, breathing, and other physiological functions are monitored. Treatment options vary and may include lifestyle changes, such as weight loss and positional therapy, or medical interventions like continuous positive airway pressure (CPAP) therapy, which involves using a A machine for maintaining an open airway during sleep.

Lifestyle Modifications:
Adopting a healthy lifestyle can often contribute to managing Sleep Apnea. This includes maintaining a healthy weight, avoiding alcohol and sedatives, and establishing a regular sleep schedule.

Sleep Apnea is a complex sleep disorder that requires careful diagnosis and management. Recognizing the symptoms, understanding the associated health risks, and seeking appropriate medical intervention are crucial steps in addressing this condition and improving overall sleep health.

Restless Leg Syndrome

Sleep disorders encompass a diverse range of conditions that disrupt the normal pattern of sleep, leading to difficulties falling asleep, staying asleep, or experiencing restorative sleep. One prominent sleep disorder is Restless Leg Syndrome (RLS), a neurological condition characterized by an irresistible urge to move the legs, often accompanied by uncomfortable sensations. This disorder typically worsens during periods of inactivity, such as when sitting or lying down, and tends to peak during the evening or nighttime.

Restless Leg Syndrome can significantly impact an individual's quality of life, as it interferes with their ability to relax and obtain sufficient rest during sleep. The sensations associated with RLS are often described as tingling, crawling, or creeping, creating an overwhelming need to move the legs to alleviate the discomfort. This constant urge to move can lead to sleep fragmentation, resulting in daytime fatigue and impaired cognitive function.

The exact cause of Restless Leg Syndrome is not fully understood, but both genetic and environmental factors are believed to contribute to its development. Certain medical conditions, such as iron deficiency, peripheral neuropathy, and kidney failure, have been linked to RLS. Additionally, some medications and lifestyle factors, such as caffeine and tobacco use, may exacerbate symptoms.

Managing Restless Leg Syndrome involves a combination of lifestyle modifications and, in some cases, medication. Lifestyle changes may include adopting regular sleep patterns, engaging in moderate exercise, and avoiding substances that can worsen symptoms. Medications, such as dopamine agonists, benzodiazepines, and anticonvulsants, may be prescribed to alleviate symptoms and improve sleep quality.

It is crucial for individuals experiencing symptoms of RLS or any other sleep disorder to consult with a healthcare professional for a comprehensive evaluation. Proper diagnosis and treatment can significantly improve sleep quality and overall well-being, ensuring that individuals affected by sleep disorders can lead healthier, more restful lives.

Narcolepsy and Neurological Implications

Narcolepsy stands as a distinctive neurological disorder, casting a shadow on the intricate machinery of the brain responsible for orchestrating our sleep-wake cycles. This enigmatic condition not only challenges our understanding of sleep regulation but also underscores the profound neurological implications that accompany its presence.

1. Disrupted Sleep-Wake Cycles:
At its core, narcolepsy disrupts the finely tuned symphony of sleep and wakefulness orchestrated by the brain. The usual progression through sleep stages is altered, leading to unexpected transitions between wakefulness and rapid eye movement (REM) sleep. These abrupt shifts result in daytime sleep attacks, where individuals with narcolepsy may uncontrollably succumb to sleep, regardless of the situation.

2. Autoimmune Factors at Play:
The etiology of narcolepsy remains shrouded in mystery, yet emerging evidence suggests autoimmune involvement. Specifically, an autoimmune response targeting hypocretin-producing neurons in the hypothalamus is implicated. Hypocretin, also known as

orexin, plays a crucial role in promoting wakefulness, and its deficiency in narcolepsy contributes to the erratic sleep patterns observed in affected individuals.

3. Hypocretin Deficiency and Daytime Dysfunction:
The hallmark of narcolepsy lies in the deficiency of hypocretin, a neurotransmitter that regulates arousal and alertness. The scarcity of this crucial neurochemical disrupts the delicate balance between sleep and wakefulness. Consequently, individuals with narcolepsy may struggle with excessive daytime sleepiness, making routine activities, such as work or driving, perilous endeavors.

4. Cataplexy: The Intricate Connection:
Many individuals with narcolepsy also experience cataplexy, a sudden loss of muscle tone often triggered by strong emotions. This phenomenon further emphasizes the neurological intricacies at play. Cataplexy is linked to the same hypocretin deficiency, underscoring the interconnectedness of the various symptoms that characterize this disorder.

5. Impact on Daily Functioning:
Beyond the neurological intricacies, narcolepsy's consequences reverberate through the fabric of daily

life. The unpredictability of sleep attacks and the potential for cataplexy pose significant challenges to professional, social, and personal spheres. Employment, relationships, and overall quality of life can be profoundly affected, demanding a multifaceted approach to managing the disorder.

6. Advancements in Treatment:
While narcolepsy poses considerable challenges, ongoing research and advancements in treatment offer hope. Medications that address neurotransmitter imbalances, such as stimulants and medications promoting wakefulness, can help manage symptoms. Additionally, lifestyle adjustments and behavioral interventions play a pivotal role in mitigating the impact of narcolepsy on daily life.

Parasomnias and Psychiatric Links

Parasomnias, a category of sleep disorders characterized by abnormal behaviors during sleep, delve into the intricate relationship between sleep and mental health. Among these, sleepwalking, night terrors, and sleep-related eating disorder stand out as phenomena with both medical and psychiatric underpinnings. The connection between these parasomnias and psychological factors such as stress, anxiety, and specific psychiatric disorders underscores the complexity of the interplay between sleep and mental well-being.

1. Sleepwalking (Somnambulism):
Sleepwalking involves complex motor activities during non-REM sleep, typically during the first half of the night. While the exact causes are not entirely clear, stress and anxiety are recognized as potential triggers. Additionally, individuals with certain psychiatric conditions, including dissociative disorders, may be more prone to sleepwalking episodes. Stressors in daily life can act as precipitating factors, disrupting the usual sleep architecture and leading to the manifestation of this parasomnia.

2. Night Terrors (Sleep Terrors):
Night terrors are intense episodes of fear or terror, often accompanied by screaming and a sense of panic. These episodes usually occur during non-REM sleep. Stress and anxiety, particularly in susceptible individuals, can contribute to the onset of night terrors. Furthermore, individuals with anxiety disorders, post-traumatic stress disorder (PTSD), or other

psychiatric conditions may be more prone to experiencing these episodes. The emotional turmoil associated with these conditions can disrupt the usual sleep cycle, making individuals more vulnerable to night terrors.

3. Sleep-Related Eating Disorder (SRED):
A sleep-related eating disorder is characterized by eating during the night, with little or no memory of the meal the following day. Stress and anxiety may play a role in the development and exacerbation of SRED. Additionally, individuals with mood disorders, such as depression or bipolar disorder, may be at an increased risk. The relationship between emotional states and this parasomnia underscores the complex interplay between mental health and sleep-related behaviors.

4. Psychiatric Links:
Stress and anxiety, as common threads connecting these parasomnias, contribute to disruptions in the sleep cycle. The bidirectional relationship between psychiatric disorders and parasomnias suggests a shared pathophysiology. Psychiatric conditions can contribute to the development of parasomnias, and in turn, these sleep disturbances can exacerbate underlying mental health issues. For instance, the

emotional toll of psychiatric disorders may manifest in disrupted sleep patterns, perpetuating a cycle that impacts overall well-being.

Hyperthyroidism

Hyperthyroidism is a medical condition characterized by the overactivity of the thyroid gland, leading to an excessive production of thyroid hormones. This hormonal imbalance can result from various causes, such as medication side effects, Graves' disease, or toxic goiter. The symptoms of hyperthyroidism are diverse and can significantly impact an individual's health and well-being.

Some common symptoms of hyperthyroidism include tremors, heightened sensitivity to heat, a rapid heartbeat, and a distinctive staring expression due to ocular effects. Individuals with hyperthyroidism may also experience sleep disturbances, including insomnia, nightmares, and night sweats. The sleep electroencephalogram (EEG) often reveals an abundance of N3 sleep, and clinicians are trained to consider hyperthyroidism as a potential cause when observing this pattern alongside an elevated heart rate in sleep studies.

Upon successful treatment of hyperthyroidism, it may take some time for sleep patterns, particularly the N3 sleep stage, to return to normal. This underscores the intricate relationship between thyroid function and sleep architecture.

In addition to hyperthyroidism, another nocturnal health concern is night-time gastroesophageal reflux (GER). This occurs when stomach acid ascends into the esophagus while an individual is lying down, leading to symptoms such as night-time heartburn, chronic cough, or chest pain unrelated to heart disease. The resulting poor sleep quality can exacerbate sensitivity to esophageal pain. Silent GER, where symptoms like heartburn are absent, can be a concealed cause of insomnia and daytime fatigue.

Assessing GER during a sleep study involves inserting an electrode sensitive to acidity into the esophagus. Lifestyle modifications such as quitting smoking, weight loss, and dietary changes (e.g., avoiding spicy foods) can help manage GER. Medications such as antacids or acid-blocking drugs are also employed in the treatment of GER.

Understanding the interplay between hyperthyroidism, GER, and sleep disturbances is crucial for providing comprehensive medical care. Addressing both the underlying thyroid dysfunction and associated sleep-related issues is essential for improving the overall health and quality of life for individuals affected by these conditions.

Addressing the underlying cause of disturbed sleep is crucial for effective management. Seeking medical advice and diagnosis is essential for developing a targeted treatment plan tailored to the specific illness causing sleep disturbances. Lifestyle changes, medications, and therapeutic interventions may be recommended based on the nature and severity of the underlying condition.

Chronic Fatigue Syndrome (CFS)

Chronic Fatigue Syndrome (CFS), also known as myalgic encephalomyelitis (ME), is a complex and debilitating medical condition characterized by persistent, unexplained fatigue that does not significantly improve with rest. This condition goes beyond normal tiredness and can substantially interfere with a person's daily life, making even simple tasks challenging.

The hallmark symptom of CFS is profound fatigue that lasts for at least six months and is not alleviated by adequate rest. This fatigue is often accompanied by a range of other symptoms, such as cognitive difficulties (often referred to as "brain fog"), impaired memory and concentration, muscle and joint pain, headaches, and disrupted sleep patterns. Individuals with CFS may experience a worsening of symptoms after physical or mental exertion, a phenomenon known as post-exertional malaise.

The exact cause of CFS remains unclear, and it is believed to be a multifactorial condition with a combination of genetic, immunological, and environmental factors contributing to its development. The onset of CFS is often associated with a viral infection, significant stress, or other triggering events, but no specific cause has been universally identified.

Diagnosing CFS can be challenging, as there are no definitive laboratory tests or imaging studies that can confirm the condition. Healthcare professionals typically rely on a thorough clinical evaluation, including a detailed medical history, physical examination, and the exclusion of other possible medical and psychiatric conditions with similar symptoms.

Management of CFS involves a multidisciplinary approach, incorporating strategies to alleviate symptoms and improve overall well-being. This may include a combination of cognitive-behavioral therapy, graded exercise therapy, medications to manage specific symptoms, and lifestyle adjustments. It is important to note that there is no one-size-fits-all approach, and treatment plans are often tailored to the individual's unique symptoms and circumstances.

Living with CFS can be challenging, both physically and emotionally, as the condition often fluctuates in severity. Support from healthcare professionals, as well as understanding and encouragement from family and friends, is crucial for individuals with CFS. Ongoing research is essential to better understand the underlying mechanisms of the condition and to develop more effective treatments that can improve the quality of life for those affected by this complex and often misunderstood syndrome.

Gastroesophageal Reflux Disease (GERD)

Gastroesophageal Reflux Disease (GERD) is a persistent and often troublesome medical condition characterized by the chronic backflow of stomach acid into the esophagus. The esophagus, a muscular tube that connects the mouth to the stomach, is not equipped to handle the corrosive nature of stomach acid. When this acid repeatedly makes its way into the esophagus, it gives rise to irritation and inflammation, forming the basis of GERD.

The primary cause of GERD is a weakened or malfunctioning lower esophageal sphincter (LES). The LES is a ring of muscle located at the junction between the esophagus and the stomach. Its function is to act as a valve, allowing food and liquids to enter the stomach while preventing the backward flow of stomach contents. However, in individuals with GERD, the LES fails to close tightly, allowing stomach acid to regurgitate into the esophagus.

The symptoms of GERD can vary in intensity, ranging from mild irritation to severe discomfort. Common manifestations include heartburn, a burning sensation in the chest that may radiate up to the throat, regurgitation of acidic or bitter-tasting substances, and difficulty swallowing. Persistent cough, hoarseness, and the sensation of a lump in the throat are also among the potential symptoms.

Several factors contribute to the development and exacerbation of GERD, including obesity, pregnancy, hiatal hernia, and certain lifestyle choices such as smoking and excessive consumption of fatty or spicy foods. Moreover, certain medications can weaken the LES or directly irritate the esophagus, further complicating the condition.

If left untreated, GERD can lead to more severe complications, such as esophagitis (inflammation of the esophagus), Barrett's esophagus (a condition that may predispose individuals to esophageal cancer), and respiratory problems due to the inhalation of stomach acid into the lungs.

Management of GERD involves a combination of lifestyle modifications, dietary changes, and medications. Lifestyle adjustments may include weight management, avoiding large meals before bedtime, and elevating the head of the bed during sleep. Dietary recommendations often involve reducing the consumption of acidic, spicy, and fatty foods, as well as limiting caffeine and alcohol intake.

In cases where lifestyle changes are insufficient, medications such as proton pump inhibitors (PPIs) or H2 blockers may be prescribed to decrease the production of stomach acid. For those with severe complications or refractory symptoms, surgical interventions like fundoplication may be considered to reinforce the lower esophageal sphincter.

GERD is a chronic and potentially serious condition that demands careful management to alleviate symptoms and prevent complications. Understanding its causes, symptoms, and available treatment options is essential for individuals affected by this condition and their healthcare providers in order to ensure effective and tailored care.

Mental Health Disorder

Mental health disorders encompass a broad spectrum of conditions that affect an individual's thoughts, emotions, and behavior, often presenting challenges to their overall well-being. Among the myriad disorders, some commonly encountered examples include depression, anxiety, and post-traumatic stress disorder (PTSD). These conditions are intricate and multifaceted, contributing to a diverse array of symptoms and experiences.

Depression a pervasive and sometimes debilitating disorder, is characterized by persistent feelings of sadness, hopelessness, and a lack of interest or pleasure in daily activities. Individuals grappling with depression may find themselves caught in a relentless cycle of negative thoughts, impacting their ability to function optimally in various aspects of life.

Anxiety, on the other hand, manifests as excessive worry, fear, or apprehension about future events. It can range from generalized anxiety disorder (GAD), which involves chronic worrying, to specific phobias that trigger intense, irrational fears. The physical manifestations of anxiety, such as increased heart rate

and muscle tension, can contribute to a heightened
state of emotional distress.

Post-Traumatic Stress Disorder (PTSD) is often a
consequence of experiencing or witnessing a traumatic
event. Those with PTSD may endure intrusive
memories, flashbacks, and emotional numbness, all of
which can significantly impact their day-to-day
functioning. Sleep disturbances, a common
accompaniment to PTSD, exemplify the intricate
interplay between mental health and physical
well-being.

One notable effect of these mental health disorders is
their impact on sleep patterns. Emotional distress, a
hallmark of many mental health conditions, can lead to
difficulties in both falling asleep and staying asleep.
Sleep disturbances may range from insomnia, where
individuals struggle to initiate or maintain sleep, to
hypersomnia, characterized by excessive daytime
sleepiness. The relationship between mental health and
sleep is bidirectional, disrupted sleep can exacerbate
mental health issues, while mental health struggles can
compromise the quality of sleep.

Understanding mental health disorders involves recognizing the interconnectedness of psychological and physiological well-being. Comprehensive approaches to mental health care encompass not only therapeutic interventions and pharmacological treatments but also lifestyle modifications that promote better sleep hygiene. By acknowledging the intricate nature of mental health, society can work towards fostering environments that support individuals in their journey towards mental well-being.

The Impact of Melatonin Secretion on Sleep Quality

Sleep is a fundamental aspect of human physiology, playing a crucial role in overall health and well-being. Melatonin, a hormone produced by the pineal gland in the brain, is a key regulator of the sleep-wake cycle. Understanding the intricate relationship between melatonin secretion and sleep quality is essential for comprehending the mechanisms that govern our natural circadian rhythms.

Melatonin Production

Melatonin production, a crucial facet of the body's intricate regulatory system, operates in close harmony with the circadian rhythm, often referred to as the body's internal clock. This intrinsic timing mechanism orchestrates a myriad of physiological processes, and melatonin plays a pivotal role in synchronizing these activities.

The circadian rhythm, inherently ingrained in human biology, is profoundly responsive to external stimuli, with light being the principal orchestrator. The ebb and flow of daylight and darkness sculpt the cadence of the circadian rhythm, acting as a conductor for the symphony of biological functions. In the absence of light, particularly during the evening and nighttime hours, the pineal gland assumes a pivotal role in the secretion of melatonin.

Nestled deep within the brain, the pineal gland transforms the environmental cues of diminishing light into a biochemical signal melatonin. This transformation is not merely a passive response; it serves as a sophisticated communication channel, transmitting a message to the entire body that it is time to transition into a state of rest and restoration. Melatonin, often heralded as the "sleep hormone," initiates a cascade of physiological changes that prepare the body for the impending journey into the realm of slumber.

The release of melatonin is a finely tuned process, reflecting the precision of the circadian rhythm. As darkness envelopes the surroundings, the pineal gland begins to synthesize melatonin from serotonin, a neurotransmitter associated with mood regulation and well-being. This synthesis is not constant but follows a rhythmic pattern, peaking during the night and tapering off with the advent of dawn.

Melatonin's influence extends beyond its role in promoting sleep. It serves as a multitasking messenger, impacting various physiological functions, including immune system modulation and antioxidant defense. Its nuanced involvement in these processes underscores its significance as a regulatory molecule, ensuring that the body operates in synchrony with the cyclical nature of day and night.

In essence, melatonin production encapsulates the elegant dance between internal biological rhythms and external environmental cues. It embodies the seamless integration of the body's intricate mechanisms, orchestrating a symphony of processes that harmonize with the celestial rhythm of light and darkness, ultimately guiding the transition from wakefulness to restful sleep.

Circadian Rhythms and Sleep-Wake Cycle

Circadian rhythms are a set of 24-hour rhythms that govern a variety of bodily functions, including sleep-wake cycles. Melatonin helps synchronize these internal rhythms with external environmental cues. As daylight diminishes in the evening, melatonin levels rise, promoting feelings of drowsiness and signaling the body to transition into sleep mode. Conversely, when exposed to light, melatonin secretion decreases, contributing to wakefulness.

Melatonin's Role in Initiating Sleep

Melatonin, often regarded as the body's natural sleep-inducing agent, plays a pivotal role in orchestrating the intricate dance between wakefulness and slumber. Its significance lies in its function as a meticulous "timekeeper" that delicately prepares the body for the transition into a restful state. This hormone, synthesized and released by the pineal gland in response to diminishing light levels, exhibits a multifaceted approach in initiating the sleep cascade.

At the forefront of melatonin's sleep-inducing mechanism is its influence on the central nervous system. As darkness sets in and ambient light diminishes, the pineal gland receives signals to commence melatonin production. Once released into the bloodstream, melatonin reaches various tissues, with a particular affinity for the brain where it interacts with specialized receptors. The suprachiasmatic nucleus, a nucleus situated in the hypothalamus intricately linked with the circadian rhythm, is a primary site for these melatonin receptors.

The binding of melatonin to its receptors, especially within the suprachiasmatic nucleus, sets off a cascade of events that synchronize the body with the natural rhythm of day and night. This engagement triggers a reduction in alertness and a gradual lowering of body temperature, both essential components for the initiation of sleep. The dimming of the metaphorical lights within the body reflects the external environment's transition into the nocturnal phase.

Moreover, melatonin's role extends beyond its immediate influence on the central nervous system. It interacts with other hormones and neurotransmitters, contributing to the overall regulation of the sleep-wake cycle. By modulating the release of certain neurotransmitters, melatonin reinforces the body's inclination toward relaxation and tranquility.

In essence, melatonin acts as a conductor orchestrating a symphony of physiological changes that pave the way for a seamless entry into the realm of sleep. Its role as a "timekeeper" not only signals the approach of bedtime but also ensures that the transition is smooth, allowing the body to surrender to the rejuvenating embrace of sleep. Understanding the intricacies of melatonin's involvement in the sleep initiation process not only sheds light on the marvels of the human circadian rhythm but also opens avenues for therapeutic interventions aimed at optimizing sleep patterns.

Disruptions in Melatonin Production and Sleep

In addition to the mentioned factors, dietary choices and lifestyle habits can significantly influence melatonin production and subsequently affect sleep quality. The modern lifestyle, characterized by high-stress levels and sedentary behavior, may contribute to disruptions in the delicate balance of melatonin synthesis.

One notable aspect is the impact of diet on melatonin. Certain foods, such as those rich in tryptophan (an amino acid precursor to melatonin), can promote its production. On the contrary, the consumption of stimulants like caffeine or certain medications close to bedtime might hinder melatonin release. Thus, dietary patterns play a crucial role in either supporting or undermining the natural sleep-wake cycle.

Environmental factors also extend beyond just artificial light. Noise pollution, for instance, can disrupt sleep by activating the stress response and interfering with the body's ability to produce melatonin. Creating a sleep-conducive environment by minimizing both light and noise exposure in the bedroom can be pivotal in enhancing melatonin secretion and improving overall sleep hygiene.

Moreover, the use of electronic devices not only exposes individuals to artificial light but also engages the mind in stimulating activities. The mental alertness induced by activities such as browsing through social media or watching intense movies can interfere with the winding-down process essential for melatonin release. Establishing a pre-sleep routine that involves calming activities, such as reading a book or practicing relaxation techniques, can mitigate the negative impact of electronic device use on melatonin levels.

Furthermore, the connection between physical activity and melatonin production should not be overlooked. Regular exercise has been shown to positively influence sleep, promoting both the quantity and quality of melatonin released during the night. Sedentary behavior, on the other hand, may contribute to hormonal imbalances that disrupt the circadian rhythm and, consequently, melatonin secretion.

Disruptions in melatonin production and subsequent sleep disturbances are multifaceted, involving a complex interplay of environmental, dietary, and lifestyle factors. Addressing these elements comprehensively through practices that prioritize sleep hygiene, promote a balanced diet, and encourage a healthy lifestyle can contribute to restoring the natural rhythm of melatonin and fostering better sleep quality.

Melatonin Supplements and Sleep Aid

Melatonin supplements, renowned for their pivotal role in sleep regulation, have gained widespread popularity as a remedy for various sleep disorders, ranging from insomnia to the disruptive effects of jet lag. The appeal of melatonin lies in its ability to synchronize the body's internal clock, helping individuals adjust to new sleep-wake cycles and facilitating a more restful night's sleep.

Individuals grappling with insomnia, characterized by difficulty falling asleep or staying asleep, often turn to melatonin supplements as a natural alternative to conventional sleep aids. The hormone, produced naturally by the pineal gland in response to darkness, plays a crucial role in signaling to the body that it's time to wind down and prepare for sleep. In supplement form, melatonin can be particularly beneficial for those facing challenges related to shift work, irregular schedules, or long-haul travel, where the body's circadian rhythm may be thrown off balance.

However, it's paramount to approach the use of melatonin supplements with caution and mindfulness. While they can be effective in certain situations, excessive intake may lead to unintended consequences. Melatonin, when taken in doses higher than necessary, can potentially disrupt the delicate balance of the circadian rhythm, the internal biological clock that regulates the sleep-wake cycle.

Inappropriately high doses of melatonin may not only fail to enhance sleep but could also result in daytime drowsiness, headaches, and even vivid dreams. Moreover, prolonged misuse may impact the body's ability to produce melatonin naturally, creating a dependence on supplementation for sleep regulation.

To optimize the benefits of melatonin supplements, it's advisable to use them under the guidance of a healthcare professional and to adhere to recommended dosage guidelines. It's also crucial to consider lifestyle factors that contribute to sleep hygiene, such as maintaining a consistent sleep schedule, creating a conducive sleep environment, and minimizing exposure to bright lights, especially in the evening.

While melatonin supplements offer a promising avenue for addressing sleep disorders, prudence in their usage is essential. Thoughtful consideration of dosage, along with a holistic approach to sleep hygiene, ensures that melatonin remains a valuable ally in promoting restful and rejuvenating sleep without inadvertently disrupting the body's natural circadian rhythm.

Strategies for Improving Sleep

NON-MEDICATION APPROACHES TO TREATMENT

Sleep Hygiene Practices

Sleep hygiene refers to a set of behavioral and environmental practices that promote healthy and consistent sleep patterns. Incorporating good sleep hygiene practices into your daily routine can significantly enhance the quality and duration of your sleep. Here are some key strategies:

1. Consistent Sleep Schedule: Aim for a regular sleep schedule by going to bed and waking up at the same time every day, even on weekends. This helps regulate your body's internal clock.

2. Create a Relaxing Bedtime Routine: Develop a calming pre-sleep routine to signal to your body that it's time to wind down. This may involve activities such as reading a book, soaking in a hot tub, or engaging in relaxation exercises.

3. Ensure that your bedroom is suitable for sleep by creating an optimal sleeping environment. This involves keeping the room dark, quiet, and cool.

Consider blackout curtains, earplugs, or a white noise machine if needed.

4. Comfortable Bed and Bedding: Invest in a comfortable mattress and pillows that support good sleep posture. The quality of your bedding can have a considerable impact on the quality of your sleep.

5. Limit Exposure to Screens Before Bed: The blue light emitted by phones, tablets, and computers can interfere with the production of the sleep hormone melatonin. Set a goal of limiting screen time to at least one hour prior to going to bed.

6. Watch Your Diet: Avoid heavy meals close to bedtime, and be mindful of stimulants like caffeine and nicotine. If you are feeling hungry before going to bed, it is recommended to have a light snack.

7. Regular Exercise: Engage in regular physical activity, but try to complete vigorous exercise at least a few hours before bedtime. Exercise can promote better sleep, but intense activity too close to bedtime may have the opposite effect.

8. Manage Stress: Practice stress-reducing techniques, such as deep breathing, meditation, or yoga, to help calm your mind before sleep.

9. Limit Naps: If you need to nap, keep it short (20-30 minutes) and avoid napping too close to bedtime, as this can disrupt your sleep-wake cycle.

10. Mindfulness and Relaxation Techniques: Incorporate mindfulness or relaxation exercises into your bedtime routine. Using techniques like slow and steady muscle relaxation or guided visualization, you can help relax your brain and get your body ready to go to sleep.

The key to improving sleep is consistency. By incorporating these sleep hygiene practices into your daily routine, you can create an environment that promotes restful and rejuvenating sleep. If sleep problems persist, it's advisable to consult with a healthcare professional to rule out any underlying sleep disorders.

Mindfulness and Relaxation Techniques

Quality sleep is crucial for overall well-being, and incorporating mindfulness and relaxation techniques into your routine can significantly improve your sleep patterns. Mindfulness involves being present in the moment without judgment, and when applied to sleep, it can be a powerful tool for calming the mind.

1. Mindful Breathing: Start by focusing on your breath.Take a deep breath and let it flow into your lungs. Let it out slowly. Concentrate on the sensation of each breath, letting go of any distracting thoughts. This simple yet effective technique can help reduce stress and promote relaxation.

2. Progressive Muscle Relaxation (PMR): This involves tensing and then slowly releasing each muscle group in your body, starting from your toes and working your way up to your head. This method helps release physical tension, making it easier to unwind and prepare for sleep.

3. Guided Imagery: Create a calming mental environment by imagining a peaceful scene, such as a beach, forest, or meadow. Engage your senses in this

mental imagery—feel the warmth of the sun, hear the rustle of leaves, or smell the fresh air. This technique can transport your mind away from stressors, easing the transition into sleep.

4. Body Scan Meditation: Lie down comfortably and bring your attention to different parts of your body, systematically scanning for any tension or discomfort. As you identify areas of tension, consciously release it, allowing your body to become progressively more relaxed.

5. Mindful Activities Before Bed: Engage in calming activities before bedtime, such as reading a book, taking a warm bath, or practicing gentle yoga. Avoid stimulating activities or screens that emit blue light, as these can interfere with the body's natural sleep-wake cycle.

6. Mindfulness Apps and Resources: Utilize mindfulness apps and guided meditation resources designed specifically for sleep. These tools often provide structured sessions to guide you through relaxation exercises, making it easier to incorporate mindfulness into your nightly routine.

Incorporating these mindfulness and relaxation techniques into your daily life can create a conducive environment for restful sleep. As you make these practices a habit, you may find that your mind becomes more attuned to a state of calmness, paving the way for a more restorative and fulfilling night's sleep.

Herbal Remedies

Herbal remedies encompass a vast spectrum of natural botanical solutions that have been cherished for centuries for their potential therapeutic benefits. Among these remedies, individuals often turn to herbal supplements to address various health concerns, and one notable area of interest is promoting relaxation and aiding in sleep.

Valerian root stands out as a popular herbal supplement renowned for its potential calming effects. Derived from the root of the Valeriana officinalis plant, valerian has been traditionally used to alleviate anxiety and improve sleep quality. Believed to interact with the neurotransmitter gamma-aminobutyric acid (GABA) in the brain, valerian may contribute to a sense of tranquility and support a more restful sleep.

Similarly, chamomile tea has long been celebrated for its soothing properties. The dried flowers of the chamomile plant, scientifically known as Matricaria chamomilla or Chamaemelum nobile, are infused to create a gentle, aromatic tea. Chamomile contains compounds like apigenin, which may interact with receptors in the brain to induce relaxation and reduce anxiety. Many people find comfort in sipping chamomile tea before bedtime to promote a calm state of mind and encourage a peaceful night's sleep.

The allure of herbal remedies lies in their holistic approach to well-being, often addressing not only the physical symptoms but also the emotional and mental aspects of health. Unlike some pharmaceutical options, herbal supplements are generally regarded as natural and, when used responsibly, may offer a gentler alternative for those seeking balance in their lives.

However, it's important to note that while herbal remedies have a rich history of use, individual responses can vary. As with any health-related decision, consulting with a healthcare professional is advisable, especially for those with pre-existing conditions or those taking other medications. Furthermore, the quality and dosage of herbal supplements can vary among products, emphasizing the importance of choosing reputable sources.

In the realm of herbal remedies for sleep and relaxation, valerian root and chamomile tea are just a glimpse into the vast array of botanical solutions available. Whether in the form of teas, tinctures, or capsules, the world of herbal supplements continues to captivate those seeking a harmonious and natural approach to promoting well-being.

About The Author

John Ray is an accomplished non-fiction writer with a passion for exploring and unraveling complex topics. With a keen eye for detail and a gift for clear, engaging prose, John Ray has established Himself as a thought leader in Self Help. His work delves into the heart of health care, offering readers insightful perspectives and a deeper understanding of the world around them.

You can find more about the author here:
https://www.amazon.com/author/John Ray

About The Author

Jay lives outside of Columbia, SC with his wife Sherry, cocker spaniel Walter and two overly-spoiled and opinionated guinea pigs, Pip and Patches.

When not working on a new novel, Jay can be found sailing on Lake Murray, working on his beloved Pontiac Aztek or somewhere on the disc golf links.